I HAVE EPILEPSY

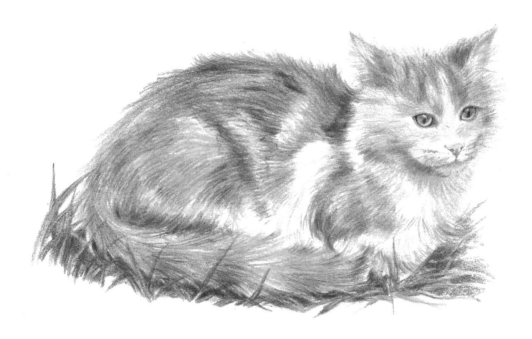

by Althea

pictures by Nicola Spoor

Published by Dinosaur Publications

I have epilepsy which means
I sometimes have a fit.

Now I take pills to stop me having fits.

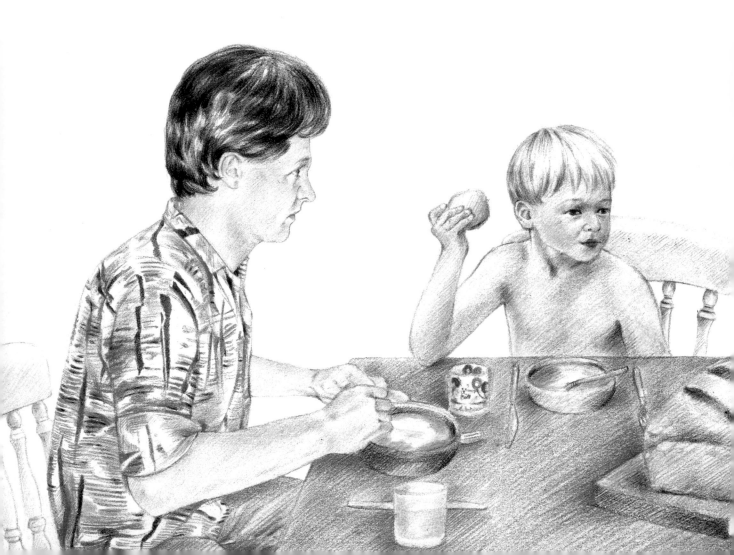

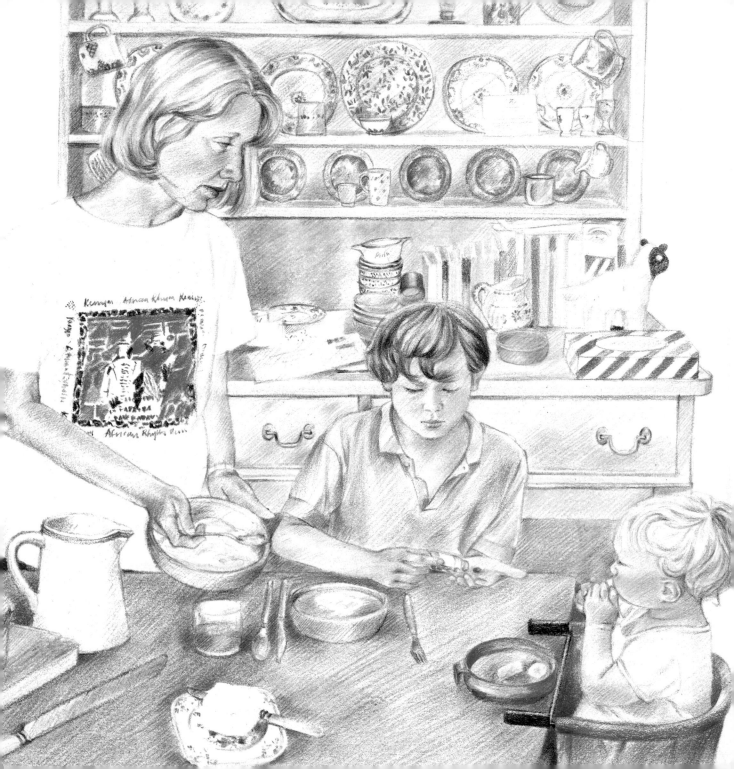

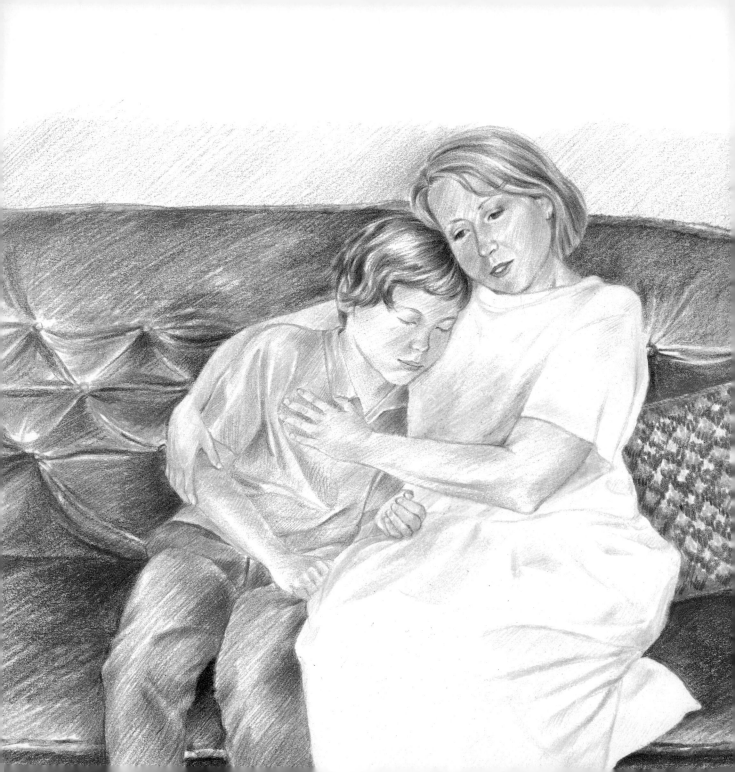

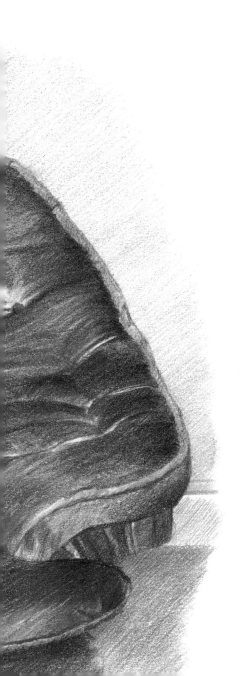

Sometimes I was a bit dizzy before
I had a fit, but often I didn't know
anything about it.

Afterwards I was very tired and
sometimes I felt sick or had a headache.
After a short sleep I felt better again.

I went to the hospital and
the doctor asked me lots of questions.
Then I did some tests for her.
She asked me to walk along a
straight line. Then she told me to touch
her finger quickly and then my nose.
She kept moving her finger which
made me start laughing. The doctor
used a bright light to look at the
back of my eyes.

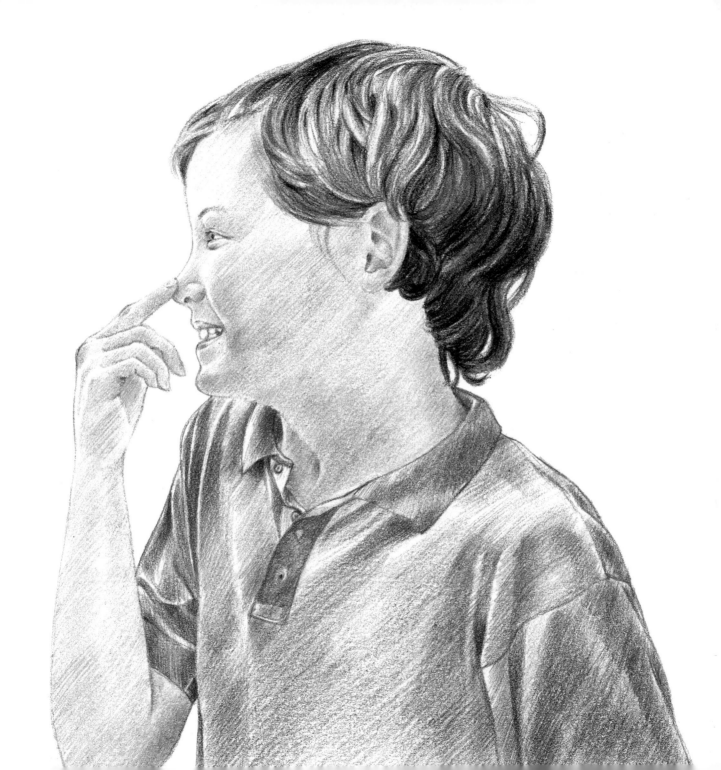

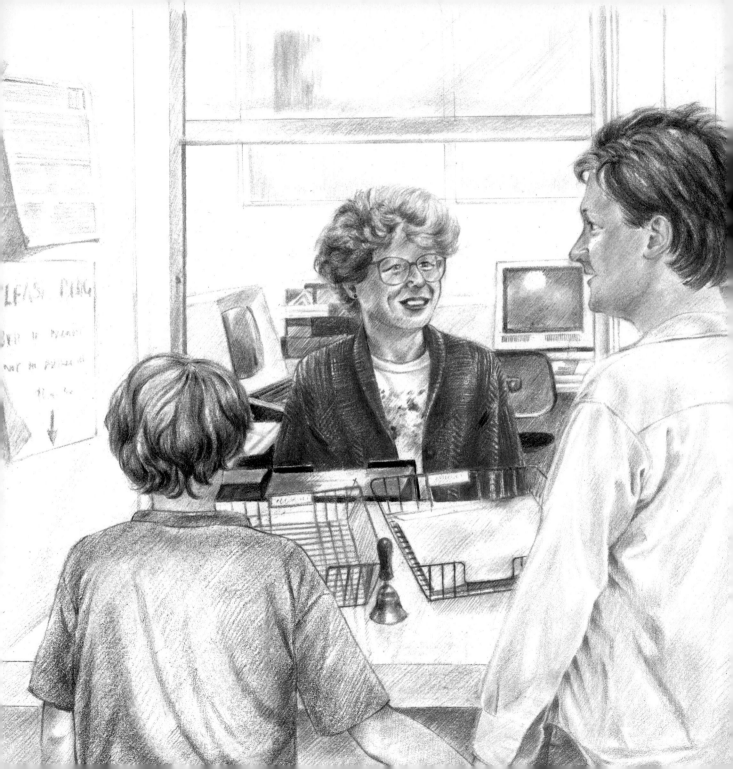

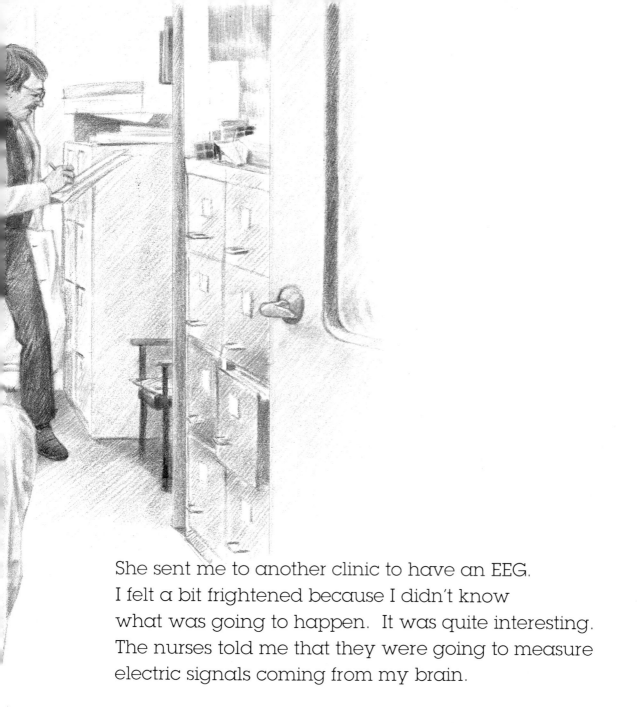

She sent me to another clinic to have an EEG.
I felt a bit frightened because I didn't know
what was going to happen. It was quite interesting.
The nurses told me that they were going to measure
electric signals coming from my brain.

They put a helmet on my head.
Then they stuck some pads attached
to wires onto my head with sticky jelly.
It wasn't very comfortable, but it didn't hurt.

I had to lie very still and close my
eyes some of the time.
I was asked to puff at a windmill
to make it go round and round.
They flashed lights on and off, too.

The electric signals from my brain
made a pattern of squiggly lines
on the paper coming out of
the machine. When we got
home, we had to wash the
sticky mess out of my hair.

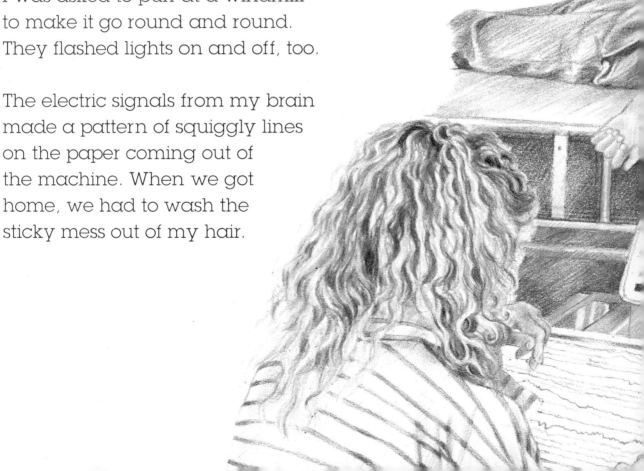

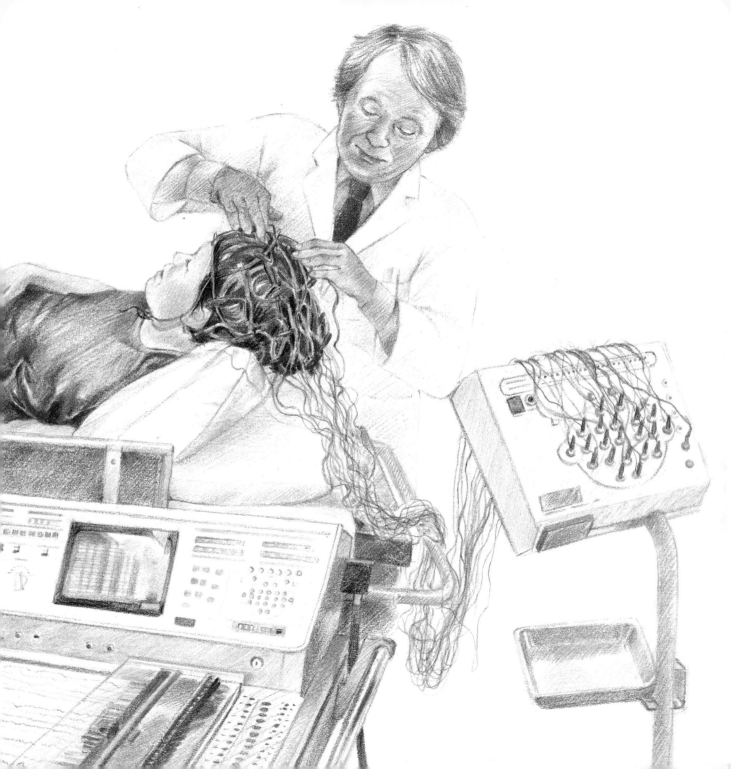

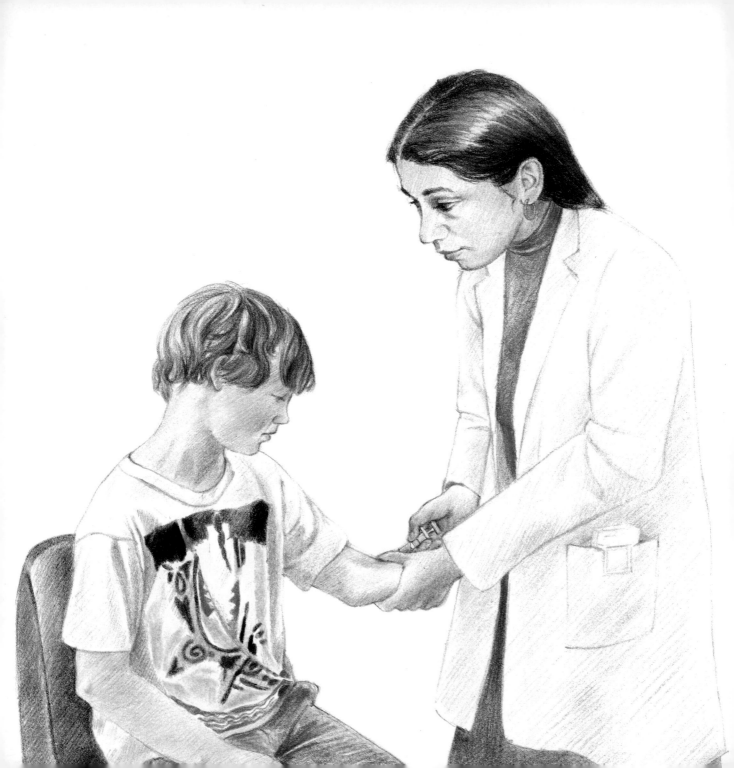

It took a while for the doctor to work out
what sort of pills I needed to stop me
having fits. I have purple and orange
pills at the moment.

I go back to the hospital every few
months to have a blood test to check that
the pills are still right for me while
I am growing.

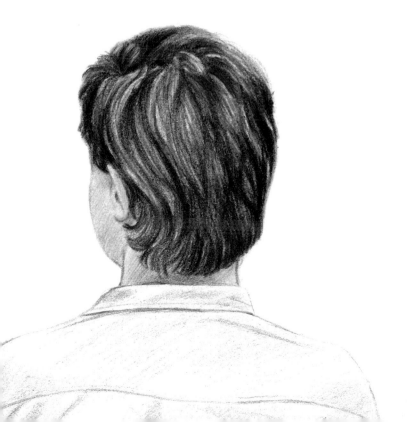

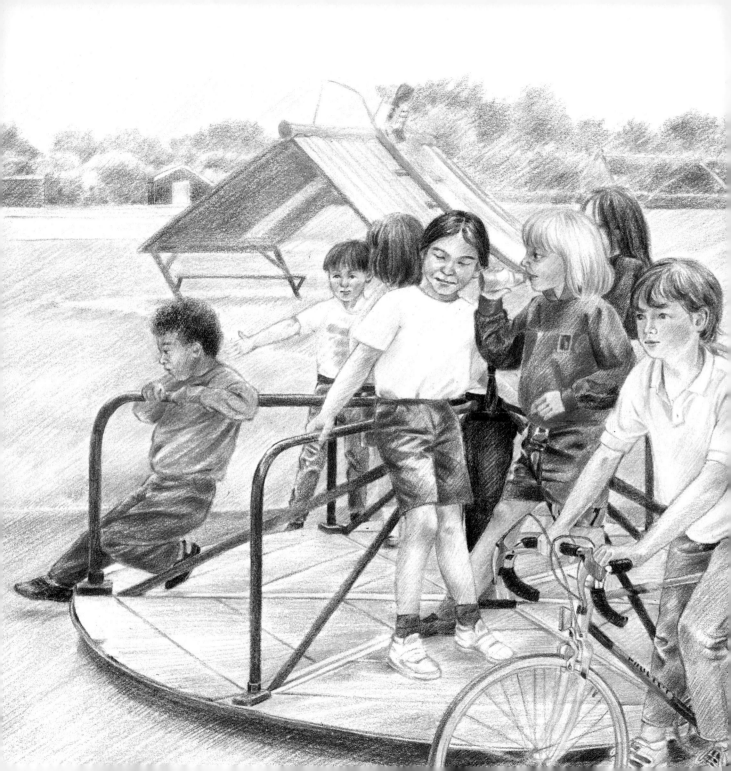

It's a nuisance, but I am not allowed to go on the road on my bike. When I have stopped having fits for a nice long while, Dad says he will think about letting me bike to my friend's house. He ought to let me because adults are allowed to drive cars if they haven't had a fit for two years.

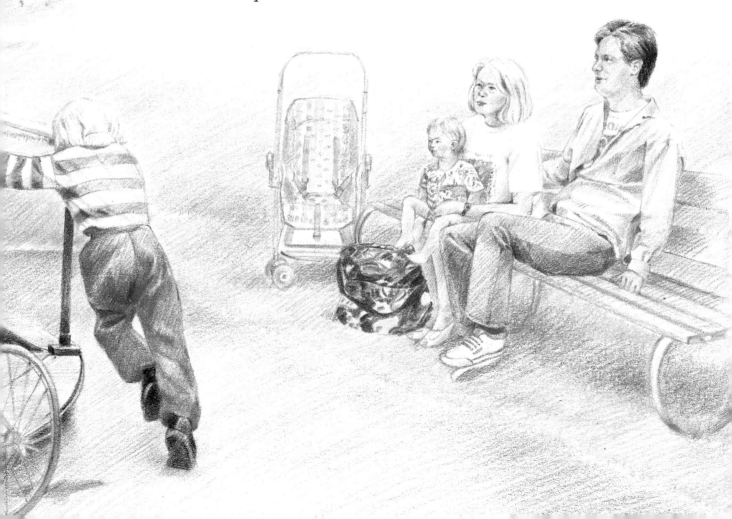

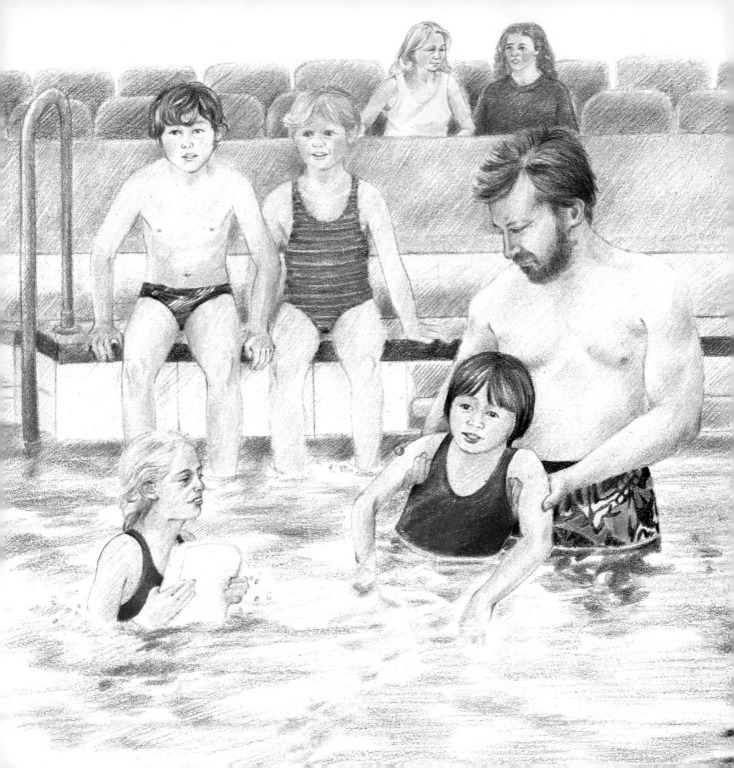

When we go swimming at school,
Mum comes to watch me.

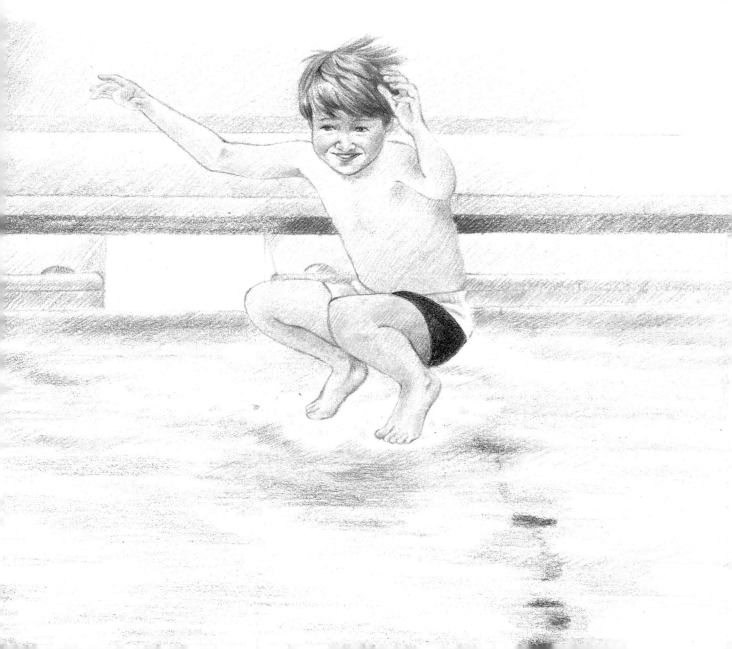

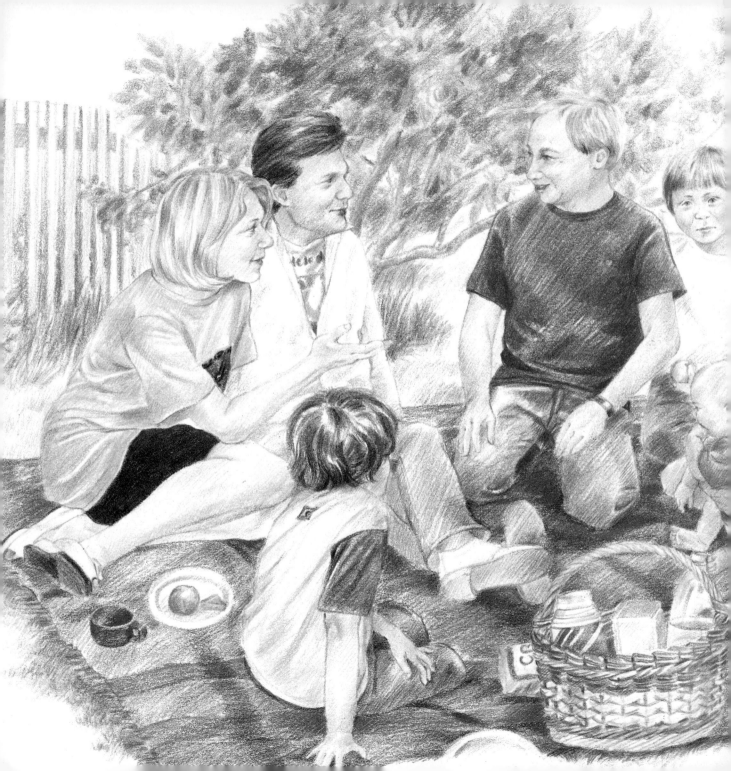

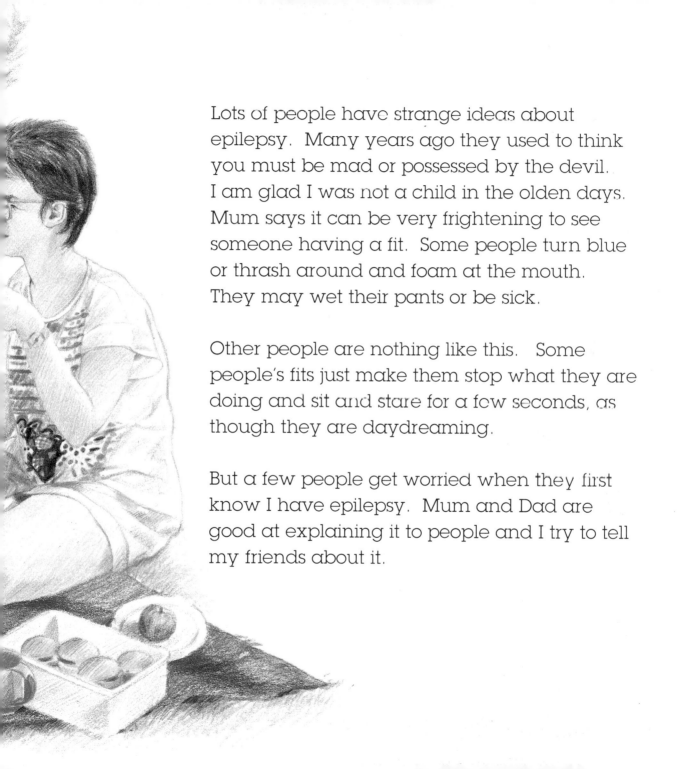

Lots of people have strange ideas about epilepsy. Many years ago they used to think you must be mad or possessed by the devil. I am glad I was not a child in the olden days. Mum says it can be very frightening to see someone having a fit. Some people turn blue or thrash around and foam at the mouth. They may wet their pants or be sick.

Other people are nothing like this. Some people's fits just make them stop what they are doing and sit and stare for a few seconds, as though they are daydreaming.

But a few people get worried when they first know I have epilepsy. Mum and Dad are good at explaining it to people and I try to tell my friends about it.

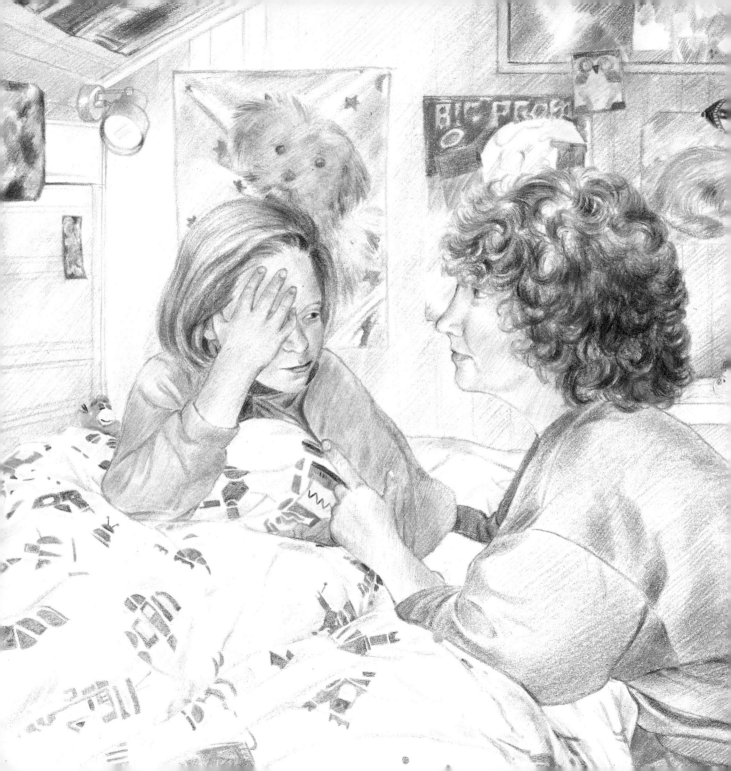

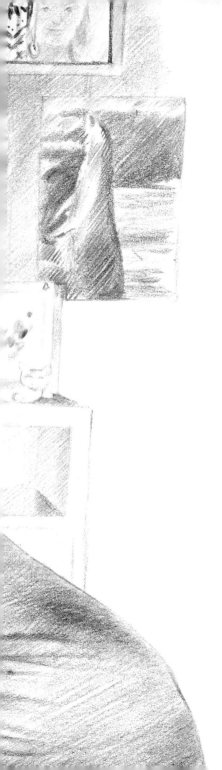

I have a friend who has fits in the
middle of the night, and she doesn't
know anything about them.
She must make a noise because
she told me her mum was there when
she woke up, and when she first
tried to talk it all came out as rubbish.
She said her fit made her feel a bit sick
and headachy, too.

I put my midday pill in my lunch box
so I won't forget to take it at school.
The teachers know about my epilepsy,
but sometimes I have to explain it to other
children. One girl even thought it was
catching.

I tell them I think a fit is a bit like
watching a programme on television when
the screen suddenly goes blank.
They tell you that there is a temporary
fault with the transmitter and your
programme will continue in a few
minutes. Then the programme carries
on as if nothing has happened.

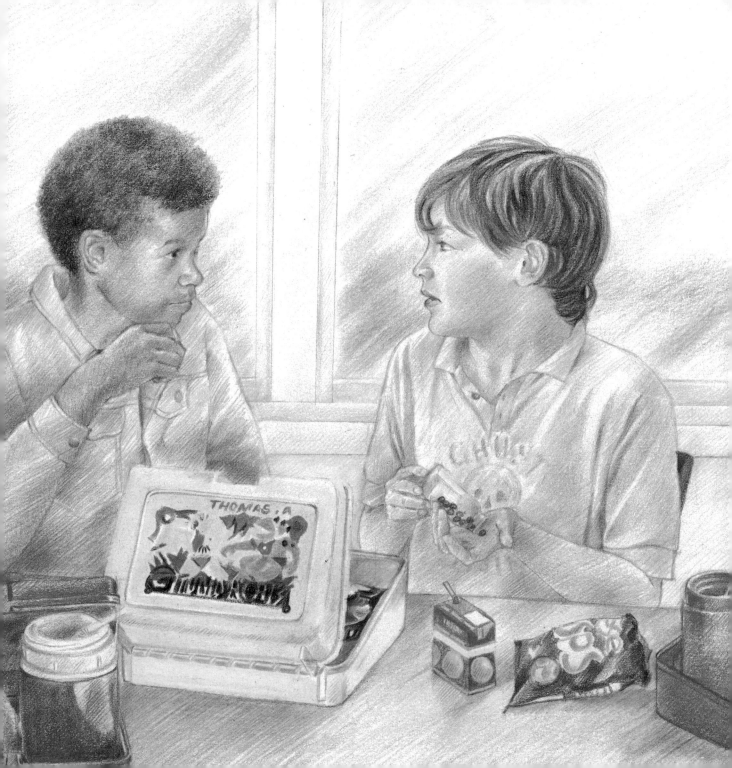

Strobe lighting can cause fits in some people, so, just in case, I covered up one eye when the lights were flashing on and off in a scene at the pantomime last year.

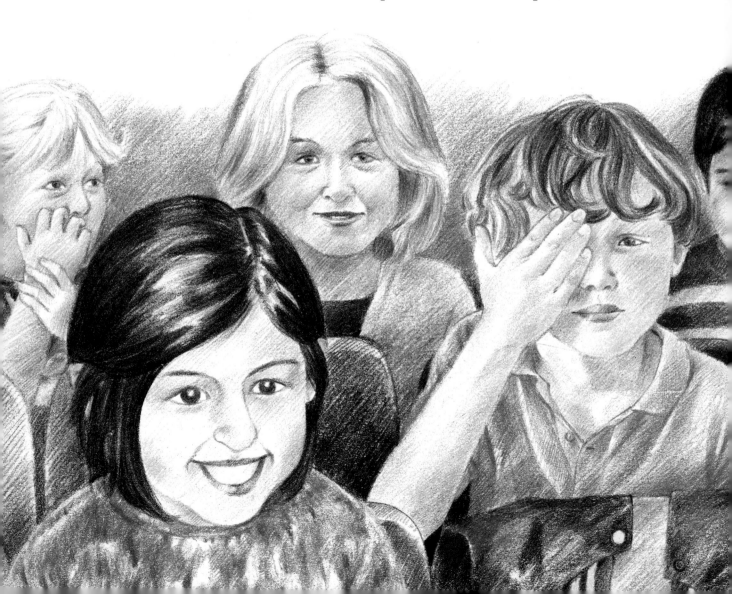

I carry a card in my pocket that says I have epilepsy, just in case I have a fit when I am out on my own. It tells people to move me away from anything that might hurt me, and to lie me on my side.

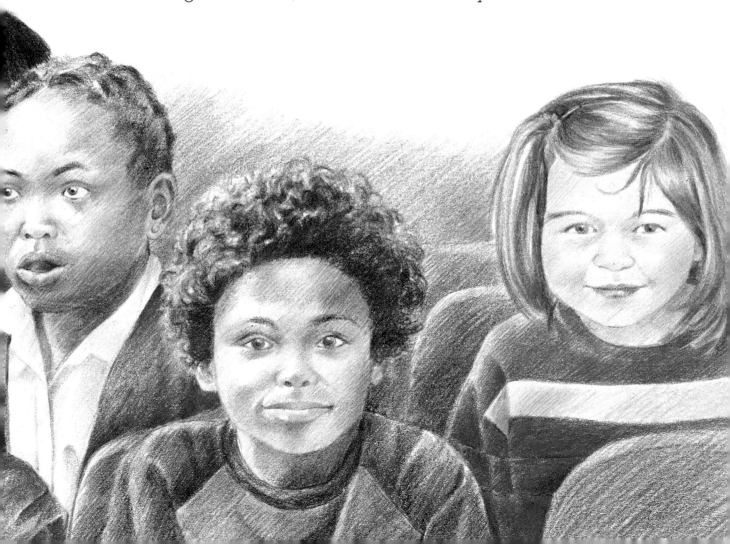

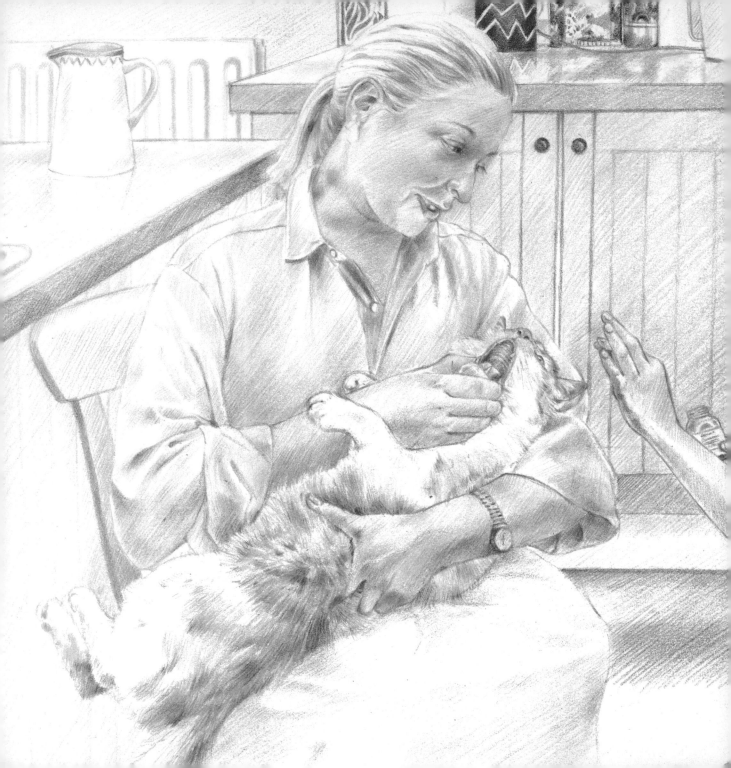

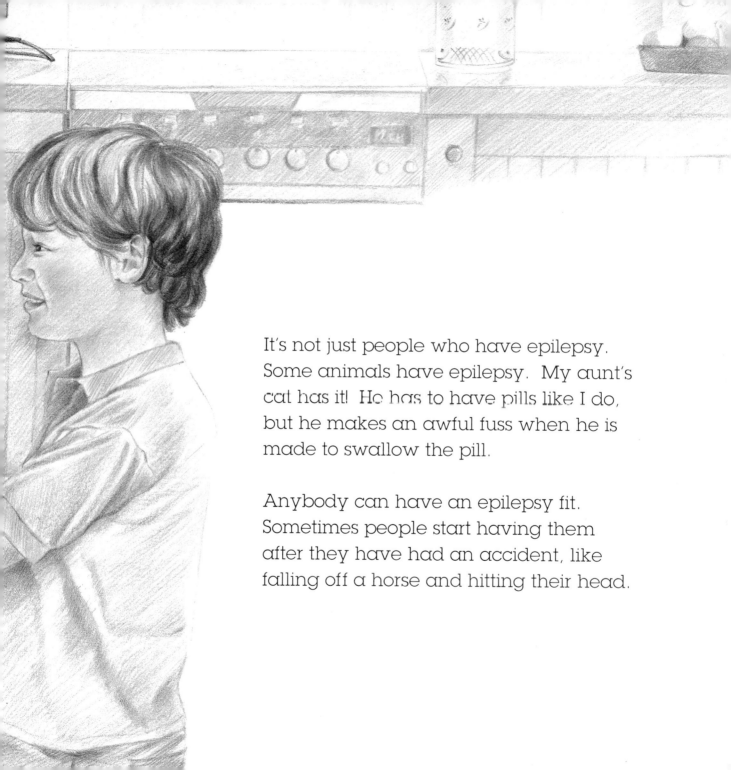

It's not just people who have epilepsy. Some animals have epilepsy. My aunt's cat has it! He has to have pills like I do, but he makes an awful fuss when he is made to swallow the pill.

Anybody can have an epilepsy fit. Sometimes people start having them after they have had an accident, like falling off a horse and hitting their head.

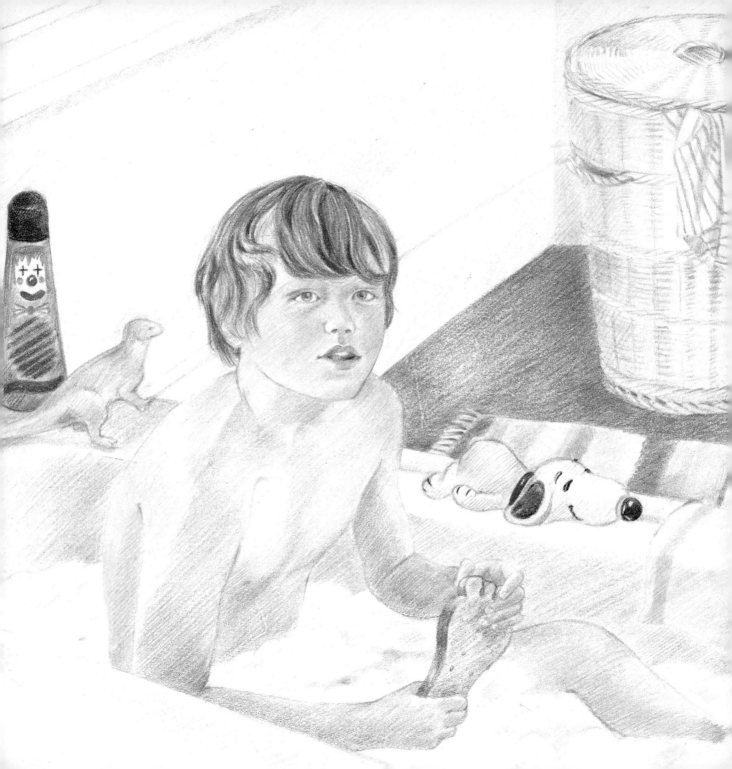

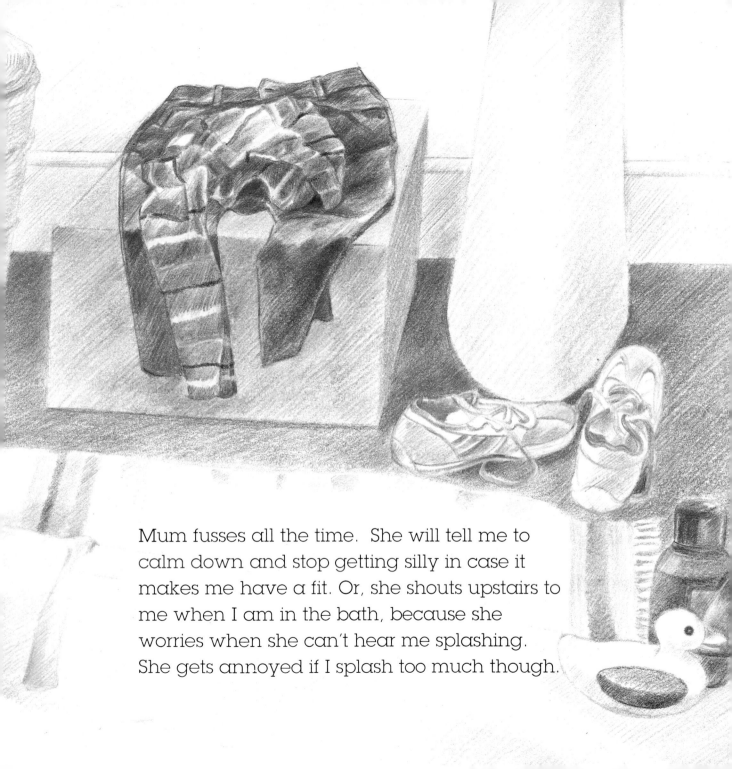

Mum fusses all the time. She will tell me to calm down and stop getting silly in case it makes me have a fit. Or, she shouts upstairs to me when I am in the bath, because she worries when she can't hear me splashing. She gets annoyed if I splash too much though.

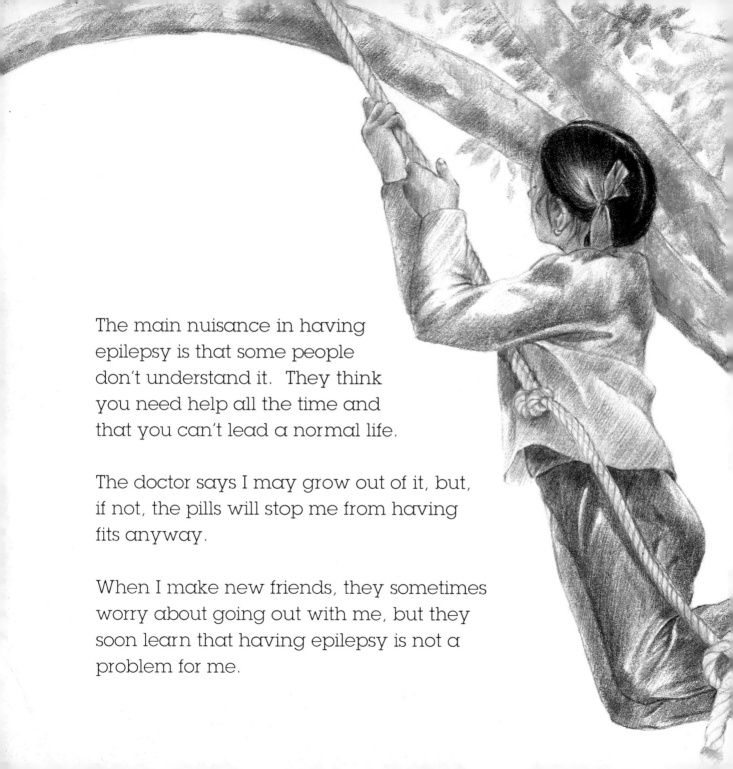

The main nuisance in having
epilepsy is that some people
don't understand it. They think
you need help all the time and
that you can't lead a normal life.

The doctor says I may grow out of it, but,
if not, the pills will stop me from having
fits anyway.

When I make new friends, they sometimes
worry about going out with me, but they
soon learn that having epilepsy is not a
problem for me.

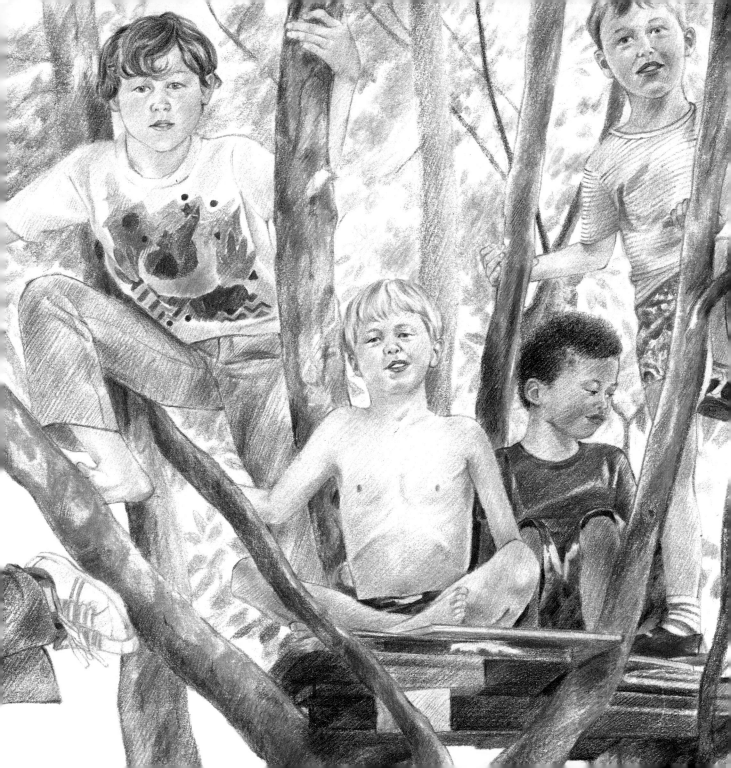

It can be alarming when someone has a fit, but try to keep calm. Move the person out of the way of traffic or other danger. Then turn the person on their side and put something soft under their head. But don't stop their body movements and never put anything in their mouth. Loosen their clothing if it is tight around the neck.

The fit may last for several minutes. Afterwards, the person will probably seem confused. Make sure people don't crowd round. Sit and talk to the person until they are fully awake.

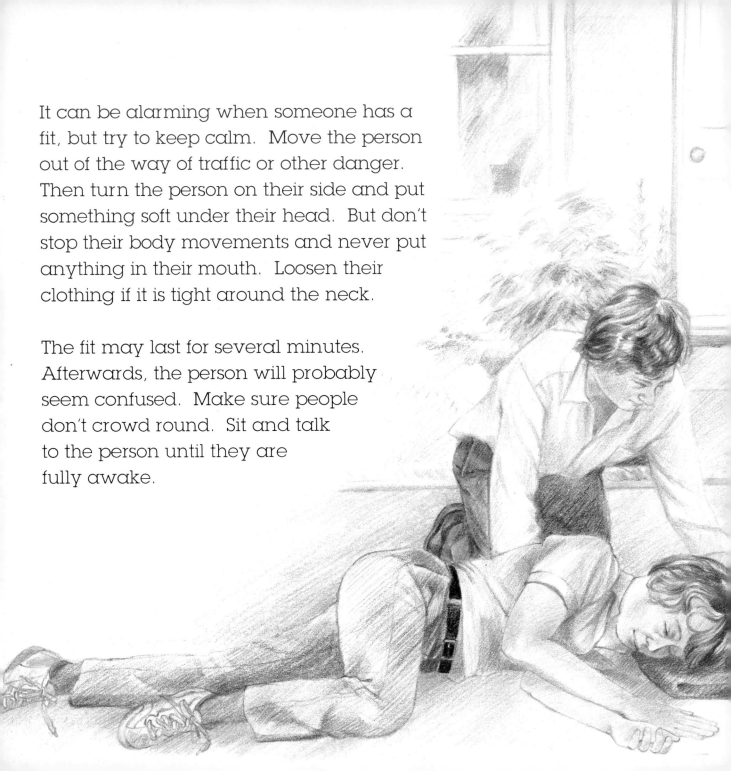